Dwijesh Kumar Panda

# Morbidity Management of Edema Leg

Dwijesh Kumar Panda

# Morbidity Management of Edema Leg

## Monograph

LAP LAMBERT Academic Publishing

**Imprint**
Any brand names and product names mentioned in this book are subject to trademark, brand or patent protection and are trademarks or registered trademarks of their respective holders. The use of brand names, product names, common names, trade names, product descriptions etc. even without a particular marking in this work is in no way to be construed to mean that such names may be regarded as unrestricted in respect of trademark and brand protection legislation and could thus be used by anyone.

Cover image: www.ingimage.com

Publisher:
LAP LAMBERT Academic Publishing
is a trademark of
International Book Market Service Ltd., member of OmniScriptum Publishing Group
17 Meldrum Street, Beau Bassin 71504, Mauritius
Printed at: see last page
**ISBN: 978-620-2-56326-0**

Zugl. / Approved by: Immunology of Lymphatic Filariasis.

# MORBIDITY MANAGEMENT
# OF
# EDEMA LEG

**Dr. Dwijesh Kumar Panda**
M.D, Ph.D. (Medicine)

# MORBIDITY MANAGAMENT OF EDEMA LEG

**Dr. Dwijesh Kumar Panda**

M.D, Ph.D. (Medicine)

# Preface

Lymphatic filariasis is a major cause of disfigurement and disability in endemic areas, leading to significant economic and psychosocial impact. It is the second leading cause of disability worldwide. Globally, 1.3 billion people are estimated to be at risk of infection. It is usually acquired in early childhood and is responsible for considerable morbidity, causing social stigma among men, women, and children. Chronic lower limb swelling is frequently encountered in clinical practice. Recurrent lymphangitis due to *Wuchereria bancrofti* infection and chronic venous insufficiency is most common. Lower extremity chronic venous disorders encompass an entire spectrum of morphologic and functional abnormalities of the venous system. The majority of symptomatic patients should undergo venous duplex ultrasonography to evaluate the nature and extent of venous reflux, which impacts the choice of treatment. Any combination of the superficial, perforator or deep venous reflux can be present. Lymphedema shares many clinical features with chronic venous insufficiency (CVI). Duplex ultrasound can demonstrate typical findings of venous valvular insufficiency. Impedance Photoplethysmography is a technique that uses optical methods to detect and measure the degree of venous reflux and the efficiency of the calf muscle pump at rest and after exercise occurring in the microvascular bed of tissue. It is a reliable, widely used, noninvasive test to detect deep vein thrombosis (DVT) in the leg (impedance) caused by blood volume variations. The blood volume in the calf distal to the cuff normally increases. However, in DVT, blood volume increases less than expected. This test is especially sensitive for DVT in the popliteal and iliofemoral venous systems.

Lymphoscintigraphy and circulating filarial antigen test reveals the cause of lymphedema. Systemic antibiotic therapy and elastic compression stocking are mandatory in both cases. Compression therapies and manual lymphatic drainage are generally contraindicated in the setting of active infection. Infection is typically diagnosed by the presence of increased temperature, erythema, and pain in the affected extremity.

**Dr. Dwijesh Kumar Panda**

# DEDICATION

A loving wife and granddaughters
Sanvi, Ani, Aishani

# CONTENTS

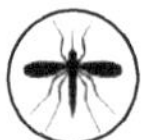

# Chronic Venous Insufficiency Resemble Lymphedema Leg

## Introduction

Lymphatic filariasis (LF) is mostly caused by *Wuchereria bancrofti* that inhabit the lymphatics and subcutaneous tissue. Infections are transmitted by mosquito vectors; humans are definitive hosts. The disease is a major cause of disfigurement and disability in endemic areas, leading to significant economic and psychosocial impact. It is the second leading cause of disability worldwide. The adult worm lives for 5-7 years. The mating of adult worms produces millions of microfilariae which are released into the blood. The major clinical manifestations include lymphedema, hydrocele in males and later stages, elephantiasis of legs. Though the disease is not fatal, it is responsible for considerable morbidity, causing social stigma among males. Massive chronic manifestations are unfortunately irreversible. WHO reports that 1.3 billion people globally at risk of LF.

Lymphedema (Elephantiasis) is a clinical condition in which there is an accumulation of interstitial fluid due to decreased lymph transport. Characteristically, chronic lymph stasis promotes both fluid accumulation and tissue changes. Defective uptake of large molecules retains water within the interstitial space and, over time, lymphstasis leads to progressive tissue changes, characterized by abnormal growth of subcutaneous tissue and intercellular matrix, and increased skin thickness. It is noteworthy that, beyond tissue fluid control, lymphatics play other important roles in tissue homeostasis, which makes lymphedema unique and far more complex than edema caused by other factors. Nevertheless, lymphedema is the most striking clinical feature of lymphatic insufficiencies, although lymphedema is hardly a disease in itself Lymphedema is best evaluated as part of a much more complex syndrome, with diverse clinical manifestations that may cause significant functional, cosmetic, and psychosocial consequences to affected individuals. Besides, some features that accompany lymph stasis may precede edema development and are an important issuein lymphatic disorders. Immune cell trafficking, and the local immune response, is impaired in patients with deranged lymph flow.

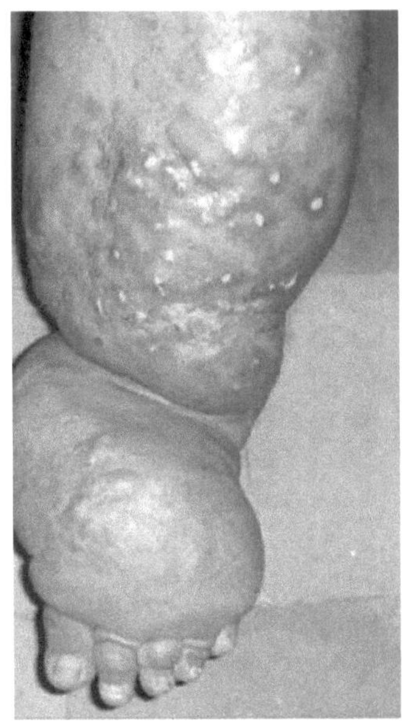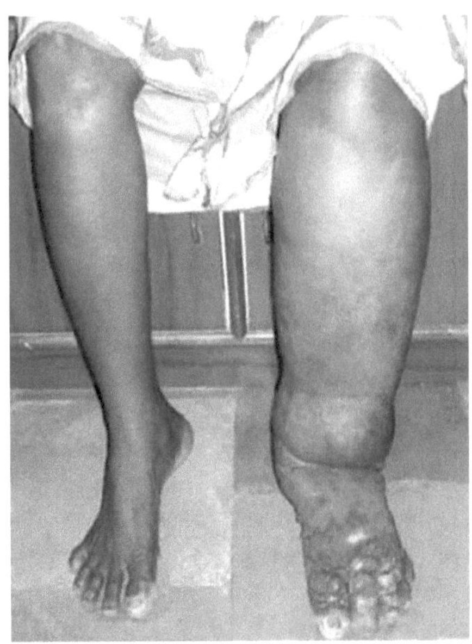

**Elephantiasis Leg**

**The life cycle of *Wuchereria bancrofti* -** The life cycle of the parasite begins with an introduction of third-stage filarial larvae onto human skin by a mosquito during a blood meal; subsequently, larvae migrate through the bite wound and enter local lymphatic vessels. Over approximately nine months, these larvae develop into mature adult worms. Female *Wuchereria* worms measure 80 to 100 mm in length and 0.24 to 0.30 mm in diameter and the males measure about 40 mm by 0.1 mm.

The adults survive for approximately five years (occasionally up to 12 to 15 years). Male and female worms mate and produce sheathed microfilariae. *Wuchereria* microfilariae are 244 to 296 microns by 7.5 to 10 microns. The microfilariae migrate into the lymph and enter the bloodstream. A mosquito ingests the microfilariae during a blood meal. In the mosquito, the microfilariae develop into third-stage larvae, which can infect another human when the mosquito takes a blood meal, completing the life cycle.

In most of the world, microfilariae are present in the bloodstream only during the evening hours, with peak numbers between approximately 10 pm and 2 am ("nocturnal periodicity"). The periodicity of the microfilariae corresponds to that of the vectors in the different regions. The interval between the acquisition of infective larvae from a mosquito bite and the detection of microfilariae in the blood is the prepatent period. In general, this interval is approximately 12 months in duration.

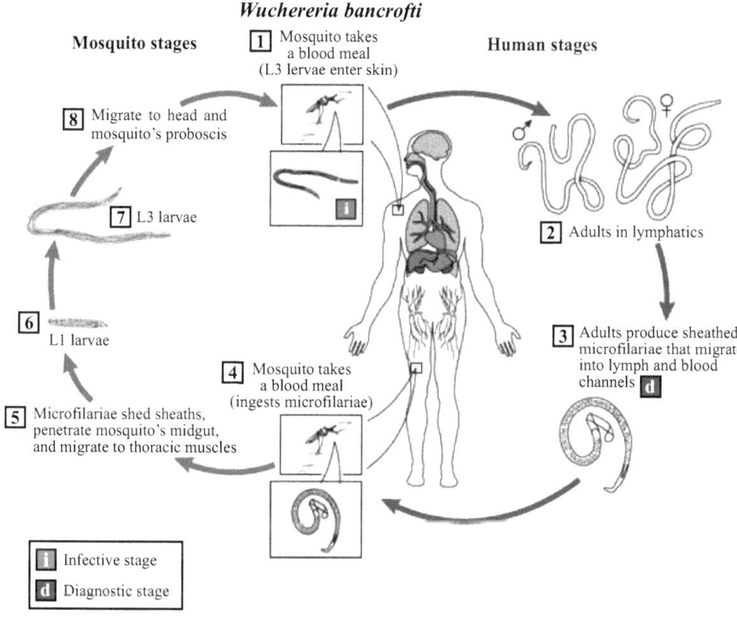


**Filarial Parasite Lifecycle**

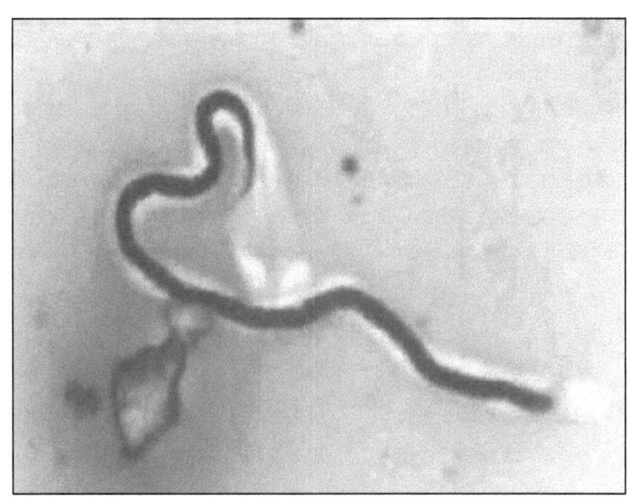

**Adult Worm**

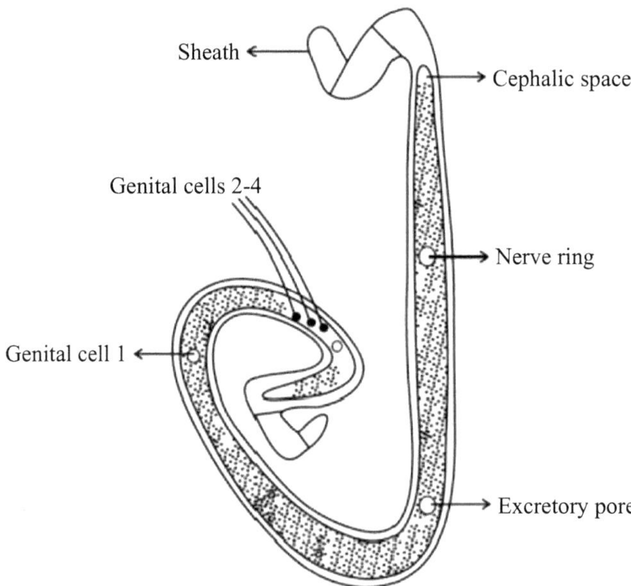



**Microfilaria**

# Lymphatic System

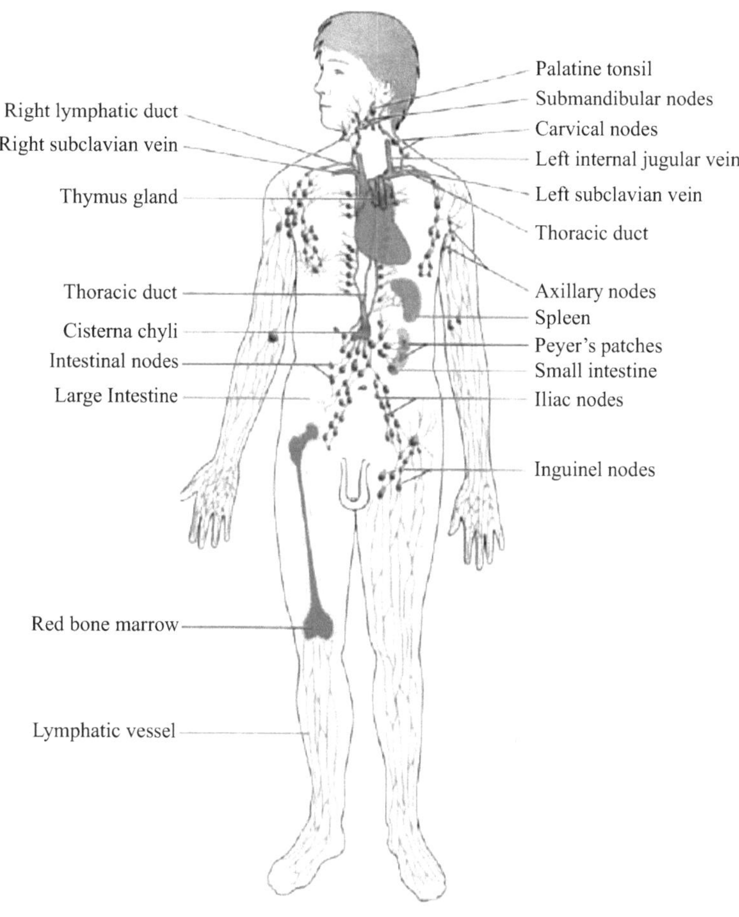



**Lymphatic System**

The superficial lymphatic system drains the skin and subcutaneous tissue, paralleling the pattern of venous drainage. The superficial lymphatic vessels drain into the deep lymphatic system, and then into the lymph nodes of the pelvis. The lymph nodes of the lower extremities consist of the popliteal and inguinal nodes.

**Popliteal nodes** – The popliteal nodes are small, deep lymph nodes located posterior to the knee, close to the popliteal vessels. They drain lymph from superficial vessels and deep areas of the leg and foot. The popliteal nodes drain into the deep and superficial inguinal nodes.

**Inguinal nodes** – The lymphatics of the inguinal region are composed of a network of lymph nodes and vessels, connecting the lower extremities to the pelvic region and abdomen. The inguinal lymph nodes are located in the femoral triangle and are grouped into superficial and deep (sub inguinal) lymph nodes.

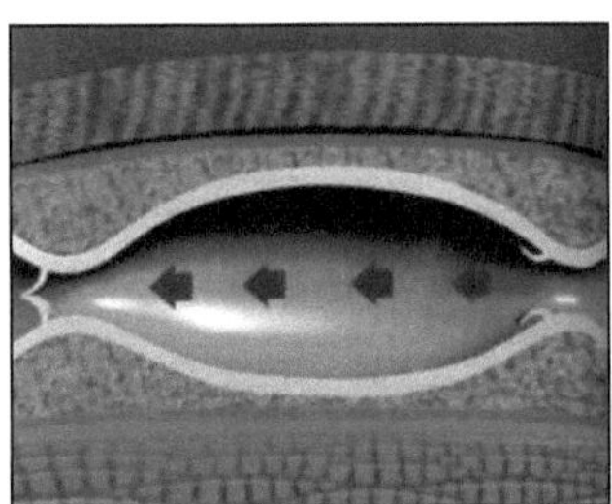

Lymphatic flow is driven by muscle contractions that produce a pressure differential to propel lymph fluid (arrows) through the system. (Couresy of BSN-Jobst.Inc.)

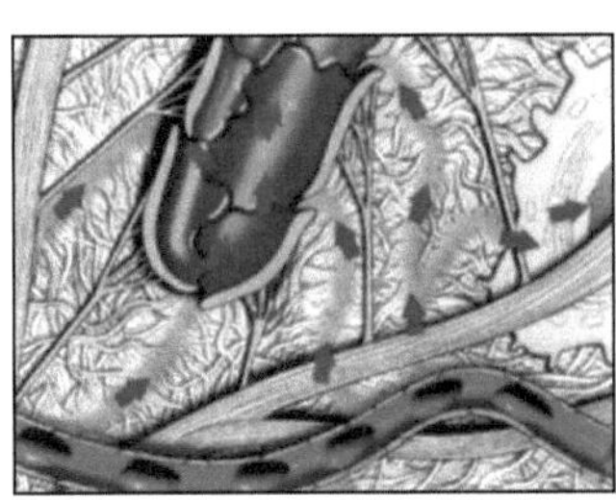

The numerous intercellular gaps that characterize the structure of the basement membrane of the lymphatic system permit flow of fluid, fat and protein (arrows) into the lymphatic capillaries. (Courtesy of BSN-Jobst. Inc.)

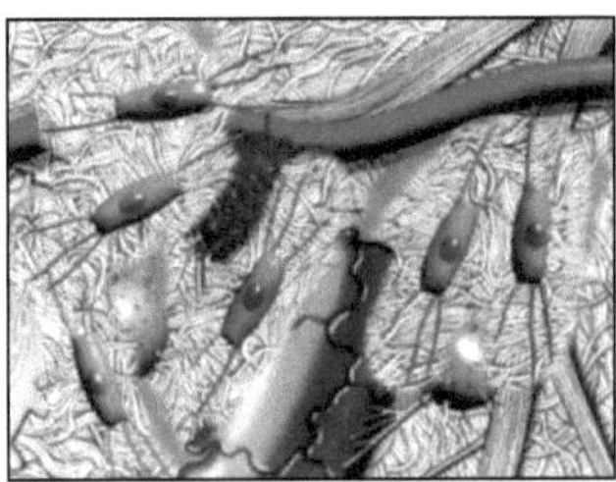

In chronic lymphedema, lymph flow is stifled, Macromolecular protein deposition increases and fibroblasts accumulate in the interstitium. Fibrovascular proliferation results in worsening brawny edema, obliteration of elastic fibers, increased collagen deposition, and fibrosis. (Courtesy of BSN-Jobst, Inc.)

The lymphatic system mainly consists of lymph, lymph vessels, and lymph nodes. Its functions are tissue drainage, absorption in the small intestine and immunity. Every day, around 21 liters of plasma fluid, containing dissolved substances and plasma protein, escape from the capillaries into the tissues. Most of this fluid is returned to the bloodstream except 3-4 liters drained by the lymphatic vessels. Without this, the tissues would rapidly become waterlogged. The cardiovascular system would begin to fail as the blood volume falls. Fat and fat-soluble materials are absorbed into the central lacteals of the villi in the small intestine. The lymphatic organs are concerned in the production and maturation of lymphocytes responsible for immunity.

Lymph is a clear watery fluid, similar to plasma and transports the plasma proteins that seep out of the capillary beds back to the bloodstream. It also carries bacteria and cell debris from damaged tissues which are destroyed by the lymph nodes. Lymph contains lymphocytes responsible to patrol the different regions of the body.

Lymph nodes are bean-shaped organs that lie along the length of lymph vessels. The lymph drains through 8-10 nodes before returning to the venous circulation. The microbes, cells from malignant tumors, damaged tissue cells, inhaled particles are destroyed in lymph nodes by macrophages and antibodies. When phagocytosis of microbes is incomplete, they may stimulate inflammation and enlargement of the node (lymphadenopathy). When a lymph vessel is obstructed there is accumulation lymph distal to the obstruction, called *lymphedema*. The amount of resultant swelling and the size of the area affected depend on the size of the vessel involved. Lymphedema usually leads to low-grade inflammation and fibrosis of the lymph vessel and further lymphedema.

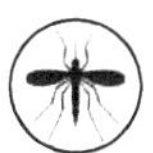

# Pathophysiology of Lymphedema

The functional unit of the lymphatic circulation is the lymphangion. Blood vessels and lymphatics are anatomically similar. The difference is in their basement membrane. The basement in blood vessels is well defined, whereas in lymphatics it exhibits numerous intercellular gaps that permit diffusion of fat and protein into the lymphatic capillaries. Muscle although highly vascular, does not contain lymphatics. The barriers between deep subfascial and the superficial lymphatic channels may be broken down with the onset of lymphatic obstruction, resulting in communications between the lymph and venous channels. In a functional state, the lymphatic system is so efficient that it can clear nearly half of the circulating albumin every day. The disease state of lymphedema occurs, when this system breaks down. Edema appears only after the lymphatic channels become fibrotic. Lymphatic load exceeds capacity, intralymphatic pressure builds, flow stagnates, and valvular incompetence occurs. Dermal backflow is seen. Fibroblasts, monocytes, adipocytes, and keratinocytes increase in the tissues. Brawny, non-pitting edema occurs from fibrovascular proliferation. The elastic fibers and basement membrane degenerate and thicken. The lymphatic channels eventually obliterated. Collagen deposit leads to further fibrosis and tissue overgrowth.

Lymphatic filariasis is the leading cause of secondary lymphedema worldwide, affecting more than 90 million people. Fibrotic changes develop with chronicity. Recurrent soft tissue infection accelerates lymphedema. Lymphatic dysfunction suppresses the local immune responses and immunosurveillance. Chronic venous insufficiency may be confused with lymphedema of legs. But it can be distinguished by chronic pruritus, pigmentary changes due to hemosiderin deposits, varicosities, and ulceration. In chronic lymphedema, edema occurs in the epifascial compartment and exhibits a characteristic honeycomb pattern on MRI and Computed Tomography. In contrast, venous edema affects both the epifascial and subfascial compartments.

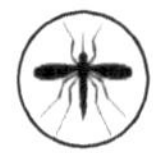

# Diagnosis of Lymphedema

A history and physical examination with typical clinical features consistent with lymphedema and asymmetric limb measurements can usually establish a diagnosis of lymphedema. Acute lymphadenitis (acute infection of the lymph nodes) is usually caused by microbes transported in lymph from other areas of infection. The nodes become inflamed, enlarged and congested with blood, and chemotaxis attracts large numbers of phagocytes. If lymph node defenses are overwhelmed, the infection may cause abscess formation in the node.

## Stemmer Sign

A positive Stemmer sign is indicative of lymphedema. It is characterized by a thickened skin fold at the base of the second toe. The examiner's inability to lift the skin of the affected limb compared with the contralateral limb is a positive sign. It is also described as difficulty lifting the skin of the dorsum of the toes of the affected limb. A positive Stemmer sign can be found in any stage of lymphedema. While it is possible to have a false negative Stemmer sign, a false positive sign is rare.

**Lymphoscintigraphy** images the flow of macromolecules and interstitial fluid from the skin to the lymph nodes, particularly in the extremities. Subcutaneous or intradermal radioactive tracers are injected in the webspace of the extremities, and imaging is performed 30 to 120 minutes after injection. The patient then performs a stress activity, such as walking for approximately 20 minutes, which is followed by repeat imaging. Criteria for impaired lymphatic function for qualitative lymphoscintigraphy include delayed, asymmetric, or absent visualization of the regional lymph nodes and dermal backflow. Quantitation of regional lymph node accumulation of the tracer appears to be more sensitive than qualitative lymphoscintigraphy. All cases missed with qualitative lymphoscintigraphy were mild grade I disease. ICG (indocyanine green) lymphangiography is one technique in which a near-infrared dye is injected intradermally. The dye is bound by albumin after injection, and uptake is therefore restricted to the lymphatics. The lymphatic vasculature can then be directly imaged with specialized sensors. Lymphatic vessel anatomy, leaking, pumping capacity, and dermal reflux can all be seen. Many lymphatic surgeons rely on ICG imaging for preoperative analysis and staging of lymphedema.

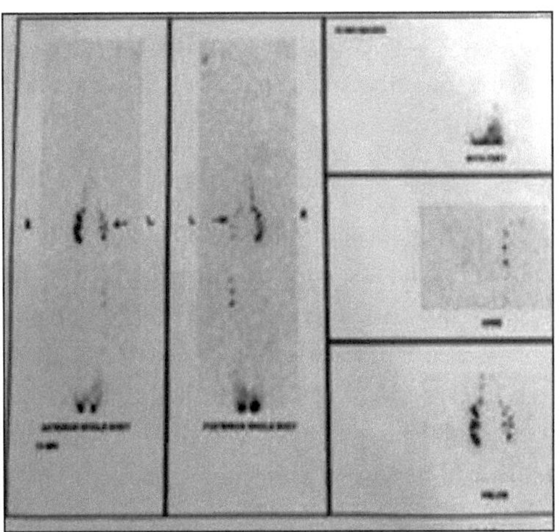

**Lymphoscintigraphy of Lymphedema Leg**

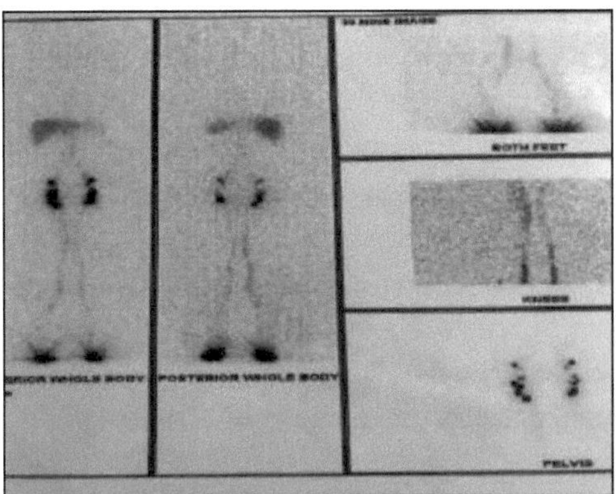

**Lymphoscintigraphy of Normal Leg**

## CT and MRI of Leg

More commonly available imaging techniques, including CT and MR imaging, can demonstrate the accumulation of fluid within soft tissues of the extremity with good sensitivity. In one study of 55 patients who underwent both CT and lymphoscintigraphy, CT had a sensitivity and specificity of 93 and 100 percent. Major CT findings for patients with lymphedema were skin thickening (95 percent), subcutaneous edema accumulation (95 percent), and a honeycombed appearance (41 percent). For demonstrating the lymphatic channels, MR has many advantages; however, the injected contrast material taken up by the lymphatics is also taken up by nearby veins. The lymphatics are typically beaded in appearance with the veins and have higher signal intensity, but the judgment is needed to distinguish them. Specialized MR techniques are being developed to exclude venous uptake, but these are not widely available.

## Serological Test

Og4C3 is a serological test based on the detection of circulating filarial antigen ( CFA) using an immunoenzymatic technique (ELISA). The wells of the microtiter plates are coated with the monoclonal antibody, IgM class of immunoglobulins produced against antigens of the bovine parasite *Onchocerca gibsoni*. This technique allows for the identification of *W. bancrofti* antigens in serum, plasma, and hydrocele fluid. It does not show any cross-reactivity with other helminthic infections (More & Copeman 1990, Rocha et al. 1996, Trop BIO 1996, Rocha 2004).

*The Og4C3-ELISA test* - The technical procedures were carried out as recommended by the manufacturers of the kit. Serological samples were processed in duplicate and the results were obtained using optical density (OD) measurement. The OD measurements for each sample were used to determine the response in units of antigen per mL (ag/mL) by comparison to a standard concentration curve for *O. gibsoni* ag/mL, included in the kit. Following the Samples with ag/mL $\geq$ 128 were considered positive for CFA.

In summary, Og4C3 showed a high sensitivity for detecting infected individuals. While the global LF elimination program is ongoing, highly sensitive and specific diagnostic tools are necessary to monitor and control the programs. There is presently no "gold standard technique" that alone is capable of offering complete confidence that infection has been eliminated. The Og4C3 ELISA presented a high performance in detecting positive individuals.

**The ankle-brachial pressure index (ABPI)** is the ratio of the blood pressure at the **ankle** to the blood pressure in the upper arm (brachium). Compared to the arm, lower blood pressure in the leg suggests blocked arteries due to peripheral artery disease (PAD).

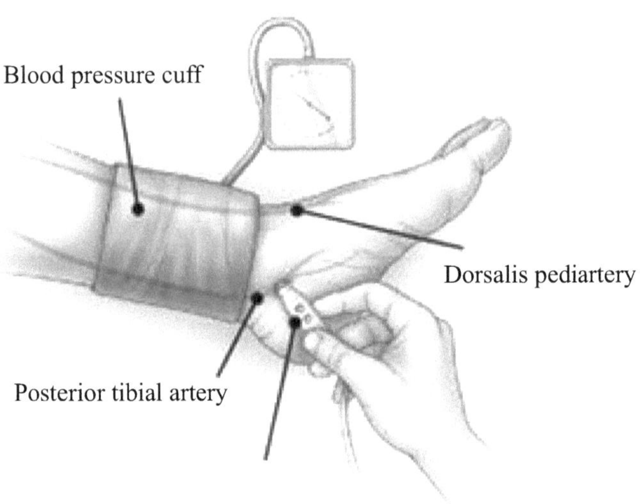


**Pressure Measurement by Vascular Doppler**

For diagnosis of peripheral artery disease, blood pressure is measured in two arteries that supply the foot using a blood-pressure cuff and an ultrasound probe.

**Procedure**

The ankle-brachial test takes 10 to 15 minutes. It can be done in a doctor's office and doesn't require any preparation other than removing shoes and socks.

The patient lies quietly on an examination table for a few minutes. The doctor measures the pressure in both arms using a standard blood pressure cuff. Then the pressure is measured in the posterior tibial artery and the dorsalis pedis artery near each ankle using a pressure cuff and a stethoscope or an ultrasound probe.

The highest pressure recorded at the ankle is divided by the highest pressure recorded at the brachial artery. This gives the ankle-brachial index. Sometimes the measurements are made before and after exercising.

The normal range for the ankle-brachial index is between 0.90 and 1.30. An index under 0.90 means that blood is having a hard time getting to the legs and feet: 0.41 to 0.90 indicates mild to moderate peripheral artery disease; 0.40 and lower indicates severe disease. The lower the index, the higher the chances of leg pain while exercising.

An ankle-brachial index over 1.30 is usually a sign of stiff, calcium-encrusted arteries. These often occur in people with diabetes or chronic kidney disease. In such cases, blood pressure should be measured at the toe, where arteries are less likely to be rigid.

The ankle-brachial index also offers information about general cardiovascular health. An analysis of studies including nearly 50,000 men and women shows that a low index (under 0.90) doubled the chances of having a heart attack or stroke or dying of heart disease over 10 years.

<h2 style="text-align:center">Comparison of Lymphedema and CVI</h2>

| S. No. | Clinical Findings & Tests | Dermato - Lymphangitis | Infected Venous Insufficiency |
|---|---|---|---|
| 1. | Pain, edema, Non healing ulcer | May he present | Usually present |
| 2. | Pigmentation of skin | Uncommon | Common |
| 3. | Stemmer Sign | Positive | Negative |
| 4. | Lymphoscintigraphy | Suggestive | Non-suggestive |
| 5. | OG4C3 Test | Positive | Negative |
| 6. | Duplex Ultrasonography | Negative | Confirmatory |
| 7. | DVT- Varicose vein | Absent | My be present |
| 8. | Diabetes and Hypetension | May be assciated | Unsully present |
| 9. | Telangiectasia | Absent | May be present |
| 10. | Ankel-brachial Pressure Index | Normal | Abnormal |

The ankle-brachial index also offers information about general cardiovascular health. An analysis of studies including nearly 50,000 men and women shows that a low index (under 0.90) doubled the chances of having a heart attack or stroke or dying of heart disease over 10 years.

## Leg circumference

Measurements of leg circumference can be taken at a particular point in the lower extremity. The clinician can use the anatomic landmarks to reproduce the measurements. The measurements can be used to classify lymphedema severity.

- 2 cm superior to the medial malleolus
- 10 cm above the superior pole of the patella
- 10 cm below the inferior pole of the patella

A difference of more than 2 cm between the affected and contralateral leg is considered clinically significant.

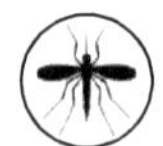

# Differential Diagnosis of Lymphedema

The main conditions associated with peripheral edema that might be confused with lymphedema are listed below.

- Chronic venous insufficiency - Lymphedema shares many clinical features with chronic venous insufficiency (CVI). Lymphedema is distinguished from CVI by an absence of typical varicose veins, an absence of characteristic skin change distribution (i.e., brawny discoloration at the medial ankle in CVI), and alleviation of symptoms and reduction of swelling with limb elevation. Duplex ultrasound will demonstrate typical findings of venous valvular insufficiency. However, a subset of patients with longstanding and severe chronic venous insufficiency may develop concurrent lymphedema.

- Acute deep venous thrombosis - Classic symptoms of a deep venous thrombosis (DVT) include acute swelling, pain, and erythema involving one limb. The onset of edema and the associated symptoms (e.g., acute erythema, calf pain) readily distinguish DVT from lymphedema.

- Post-thrombotic syndrome - Post-thrombotic syndrome (PTS) is the development of chronic venous symptoms and/or signs secondary to DVT. These include pain, venous dilation, edema, pigmentation, skin changes, and venous ulcers. A prior history of DVT can distinguish this condition from lymphedema.

- Limb hypertrophy – Several syndromes are characterized by limb size discrepancies that may be due to hypertrophy of the soft tissue and bones (ie, Klippel-Trenaunay syndrome), or overgrowth of body parts in a disproportionate fashion (i.e., Proteus syndrome), that may affect one or more limbs. These syndromes are associated with other clinical manifestations, such as capillary malformations, which may help to distinguish them from lymphedema.

- Lipedema - Lipedema is a rare adipose disorder characterized as the abnormal deposition of fat with associated edema.Pedigree analysis suggests it is inherited as an X-linked dominant or autosomal dominant condition. It occurs almost exclusively in women. Patients with lipedema may have family members who also have abnormal patterns of fat deposition but will generally not have a history of lymph node resection or trauma as seen with lymphedema. Patients with lipedema may complain of pain and tenderness and sustain easy bruising. Elevating the limbs has no effect on limbs with lipedema. The feet are usually not involved with lipedema, but the feet may or may not be involved in lymphedema. A physical examination will help differentiate lipedema from lymphedema; patients with lipedema will not generally have pitting edema while lymphedema may have pitting edema. If a question remains, imaging studies may help. Patients with lipedema usually have the normal lymphatic function, whereas patients with lymphedema may have dermal backflow and lack of uptake in lymph nodes.

- Myxedema - Myxedema results from infiltration of the skin by glycosaminoglycans with associated water retention leading to nonpittings edema. The serum TSH is elevated, whereas serum free T4 is low. Iodine deficiency is the most common cause. The symptoms may include cold intolerance, modest weight gain, due to fluid retension, coarse skin, and facial puffiness due to infiltration with mucopolysaccharides and proteinaccous ground substance.

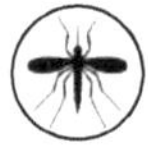

# Treatment of Lymphatic Filariasis and Lymphedema

The approach to the treatment of lymphatic filariasis requires an understanding of the antimicrobial agent and the possibility of coinfection. The treatment of choice for lymphatic filariasis is diethylcarbamazine (DEC). Patients with lymphatic filariasis should receive single-dose treatment with DEC (6 mg/kg). Doxycycline has macrofilaricidal activity and reduces pathology in mild to moderate disease. In areas where lymphatic filariasis is endemic, management consists of a three-drug combination regimen consisting of ivermectin, diethylcarbamazine, and albendazole (single dose). Lymphedema patients should wash affected areas twice daily, use antibacterial creams on small abrasions, keep nails clean, and wear shoes. The affected limb should be exercised regularly to promote lymph flow and should be elevated at night. Complex decongestive physiotherapy can also be effective in some cases. All episodes of cellulitis should be treated. Antibiotics that have adequate coverage for gram-positive cocci should be promptly administered for cellulitis. Severe cellulitis, lymphangitis, or bacteremia requires intravenous antibiotics. If patients experience three or more episodes of cellulitis in a year, an extended period of oral antibiotic therapy is suggested. All patients with severe lymphedema should follow the general measures, intensive physiotherapy, complete decongestive therapy and use of pneumatic compression devices.

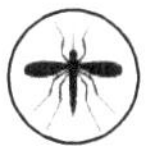

# Surgical Options

Lymphovenous bypass surgical procedures are effective in patients with early-stage lymphedema. Excisional procedures for lymphedema aim to remove the fibro-fatty tissue that is deposited below the skin. Radical excision of skin and subcutaneous tissues is generally reserved for patients with very severe disease who have failed all other measures. Surgical therapy for lymphedema is largely disappointing. Outcome after operative intervention in the lower extremity is unfavorable.

**Nonoperative measures -** The compressive garments and decongestive therapy are the initial approach for the management of lymphedema.

The indications for operative management of primary and secondary lymphedema include :

- Localized primary lesions (including microcystic and macroscopic lymphatic malformations)
- Failed nonoperative management
- Recurrent cellulitis
- Leakage of lymph into body cavities, organs, or externally
- Limitation of function
- Deformity or disfigurement
- Pain
- Diminished quality of life, including emotional and psychosocial distress.

The goals of surgical management of lymphedema are to alleviate pain and discomfort, retain or restore function, reduce the risk of infection, prevent disease progression, improve cosmesis, and limit deformity.

There is no consensus on the timing of surgery or optimal surgical intervention. The decision to perform an operative procedure to treat lymphedema should be made on a case-by-case basis.

For patients who will undergo a physiologic procedure, venous duplex ultrasound is performed to rule out venous thrombosis, venous insufficiency, and/or valvular incompetence.

**Lymphatic bypass procedures** - Lymphatic bypass procedures are used in the following settings:

- Failure of nonoperative management
- Recurrent cellulitis or lymphangitis
- Dissatisfaction with compression garments or impaired quality of life

**Contraindications to lymphatic bypass procedures include:**

- Extensive tissue fibrosis
- Late-stage lymphedema changes
- Venous hypertension
- Patient noncompliance with compression therapy or postoperative care plans

The lymphatic bypass procedures are categorized as lymphatic-lymphatic bypass and lymphovenous bypass procedures.

The basic principle is that the lymphatic vessels distal to the lymphatic obstruction are anastomosed to healthy lymphatic vessels or veins proximal to the obstruction.

An alternative technique involves using a vein graft harvested from another anatomic site and used as the conduit between transected lymphatic vessels and a draining regional vein.

**Methods** - There are several methods used to perform a bypass procedure. There is no consensus for the specific type of lymphatic bypass procedure to be performed.

**Lymphatic-lymphatic bypass** - Lympholymphatic bypass transfers soft tissue resected from an unaffected site to a site that is proximal to that affected by lymphedema and followed by a direct anastomosis of the lymphatic vessels. collecting lymphatics are identified and microsurgically anastomosed to the donor lymphatics.

**Lymphovenous bypass** - Lymphovenous bypass is an alternative to the lymphatic-lymphatic technique. A vein interposition graft is used to connect the distal lymphatic vessels with vessels proximal to the obstruction. Proximal vessels used in this technique include lymphatic vessels, adjacent veins, or deeper and larger veins. Multiple lymphatic vessels can be anastomosed to the vein graft.

**Lymphaticovenular anastomosis** - This is a supermicrosurgical technique used to anastomose distal subdermal lymphatic vessels and adjacent venules less than 0.8 mm in diameter.

**Outcomes** - Most of the outcome data for physiologic techniques are from retrospective reviews of mostly lymphatic bypass procedures. Lymphatic bypass procedures result in highly variable responses, ranging from a complete response to none.

Management of secondary lymphedema is typically nonsurgical  The decision to perform an operative procedure to treat lymphedema should be made on a case-by-case basis

The physiologic procedures create new channels to increase the capacity of the lymphatic system to transport lymph fluid. The basic principle is that the lymphatic vessels distal to the lymphatic obstruction are anastomosed to healthy lymphatic vessels or veins proximal to the obstruction.

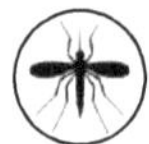

# Chronic Venous Insufficiencies

**Anatomy and Pathophysiology of CVI**

Superficial, deep, and perforating veins are the three distinct networks of venous drainage of the lower extremity. Telangiectasias and reticular veins may be symptomatic, most are asymptomatic, and patients often find the cosmetic appearance of their veins distressing. The greater and lesser saphenous veins lie in the subcutaneous plane without having an arterial counterpart. The deep veins of the leg lie in the subfascial layer. They are popliteal, femoral veins account for 85 to 90% of venous drainage of the leg. The perforating veins connect the superficial and deep venous systems. All leg veins have bicuspid valves that permit only cephalic directional blood flow. Hydrostatic pressure in the standing posture is approximately 80 mm Hg at rest. The deep veins are compressed by the contraction of leg musculature during movement. The pressure in the deep veins rises, and blood is propelled proximally. Retrograde flow into the superficial system is prevented by closure of the venous valves. A diseased venous system or compromised muscle pump can lead to venous insufficiency. In valvular incompetence, the venous pressure in the deep remains high. The tissues are exposed to elevated venous pressures. This results in venous hypertension or chronic venous insufficiency. Hypertension in the deep system is transmitted to superficial veins and results in edema. Lipodermatosclerosis develop due to changes in the skin and subcutaneous tissues. Inflammation and tender erythematous induration are seen proximal to the medial malleolus of the ankle. The skin develops pigmentary changes and fibrosis in the subcutaneous tissues. Lipodermatosclerosis leads to venous ulceration and impairment of wound healing. Patients with congestive heart failure, hepatic congestion, and lymphedema do not routinely develop skin changes and ulcerations typical of venous disease. Inflammation and venous hypertension lead to leukocyte plugging in the skin capillaries resulting in the release of a cascade of cytokines, free radicals, and proteolytic enzymes such as collagenase which might predispose to ulceration.

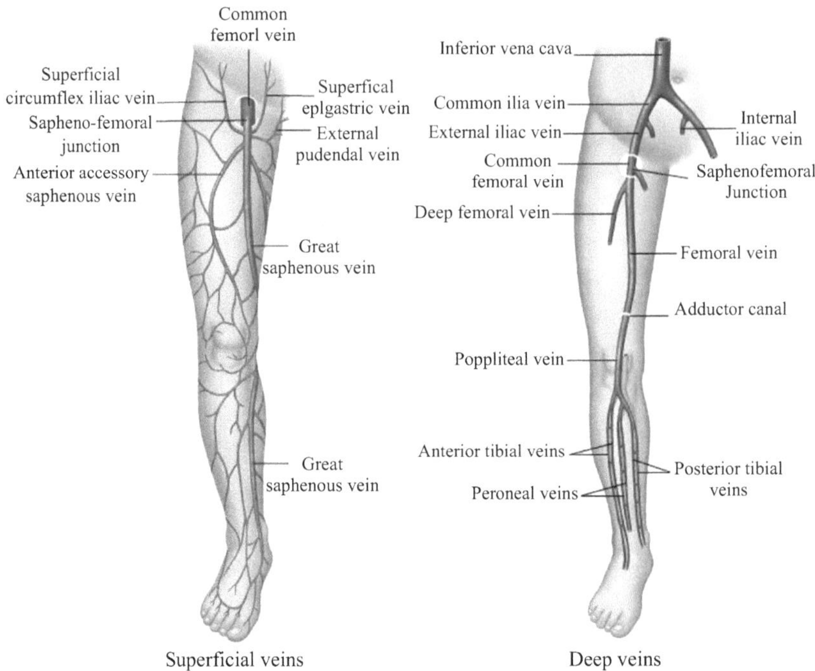


**Venous System of Lower Extremity**

**Epidemiology and Risk Factors**

Chronic vein abnormalities are present in up to 50 percent of individuals. Epidemiologic studies are generally limited to either those with mild abnormalities (telangiectasias, reticular veins), uncomplicated varicose veins with or without venous reflux, or longstanding venous insufficiency (skin changes, venous ulceration).

**Risk factors -** The risk factors for developing the chronic venous disease include advancing age, family history of venous disease, ligamentous laxity (hernia, flat feet), prolonged standing, increased body mass index, smoking, sedentary lifestyle, lower extremity trauma, prior venous thrombosis, high estrogen states, and pregnancy. The proportion of the population suffering from obesity and chronic venous insufficiency is increasing, and obese patients are more likely to be symptomatic as a result of their venous disease.

Despite the well-known association, a history of deep venous thrombosis is obtained in less than one-third of patients with severe clinical manifestations of chronic venous disease.  Duplex ultrasound in these patients may identify valvular insufficiency, chronic vein wall thickening, or chronic thrombosis indicative of post-thrombotic syndrome. Prevalence rates appear to be lower in non-Western populations. The Western lifestyle such as prolonged standing and sitting increases the likelihood of developing chronic venous disease.

**Chronic Venous Insufficiencies**

Chronic venous insufficiencies are the wide spectrum of vein abnormalities such as venous dilation and venous reflux of long duration. The symptoms include a wide range of clinical signs of superficial venous dilation to chronic changes with ulceration. Inadequate muscle pump function, incompetent venous pressure (reflux), venous thrombosis or stenosis are causes of venous hypertension. These abnormalities are present in up to 50 percent of individuals. The risk factors of the disease include advanced age, family history of venous disease, hernia, flat feet, prolong standing, increase body mass index, smoking, sedentary lifestyle, lower extremity trauma, post-thrombotic, hereditary conditions, high estrogen states, and pregnancy. Duplex ultrasound identifies valvular insufficiency, vein wall thickening or chronic thrombosis. Prolonged standing and sitting increase the incidence of developing chronic venous disease.

Lower extremity ulceration and swelling are the most common presentations of patients seeking medical attention. Venous ulcers referred to as "stasis ulcers" are seen in 80 to 90% of ulcers in the leg. It carries a significant impact on the patient's quality of life and economic productivity. It is less likely than an arterial disease to lead to limb threat. It is estimated that approximately 1 in 1000 people have an unhealed venous leg ulcer. Several factors contribute to venous ulcers. A history of prior trauma or phlebitis, family history of varicose veins, obesity, diabetes and genetic component of the disease will increase the development of CVI. Heart failure, hypertension, renal disease, and rheumatoid arthritis are additional causes. It is more common in women. Chronic pain is a complaint of two-thirds of patients with venous ulceration. It also increases with the increase of age (peak occurrence at 60 to 80 years).

The average duration of most ulcers is longer than 1 year. Ulceration lasts more than 5 years. The recurrence rate of ulceration is nearly 75%. An estimated 2 million workdays are lost annually in the United States because of leg ulcers alone.

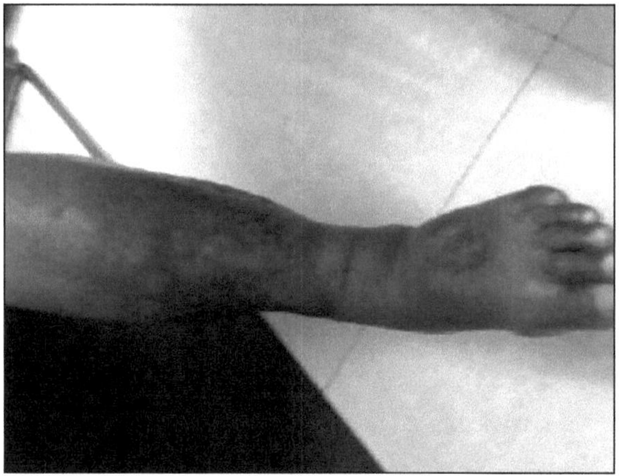

**CVI Leg-Healed Ulcer**

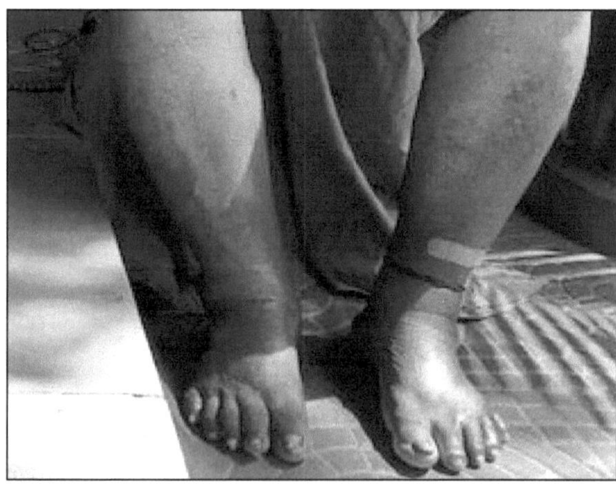

**CVI Leg-Acute Ulcer**

Chronic vein abnormalities are present in up to 50 percent of individuals. Venous claudication, which is severe deep pain and tightness typically in the thigh muscles with vigorous exercise, can occur in the setting of longstanding venous obstruction. Visible clinical signs of chronic venous disorders in increasing severity include dilated veins (telangiectasia, varicose veins), leg edema, skin changes (lipodermatosclerosis; a fibrosing dermatitis of the subcutaneous tissue), and skin ulceration. The prevalence of symptoms and clinical signs of venous disease correlates with the presence of venous reflux (superficial, deep) identified with duplex ultrasound. The diagnosis of chronic venous disease is suggested by the presence of typical symptoms (leg pain, fatigue, heaviness), physical examination findings, the presence of venous reflux (superficial, deep), which is diagnosed by duplex ultrasound based on the duration of reversed (retrograde) flow.

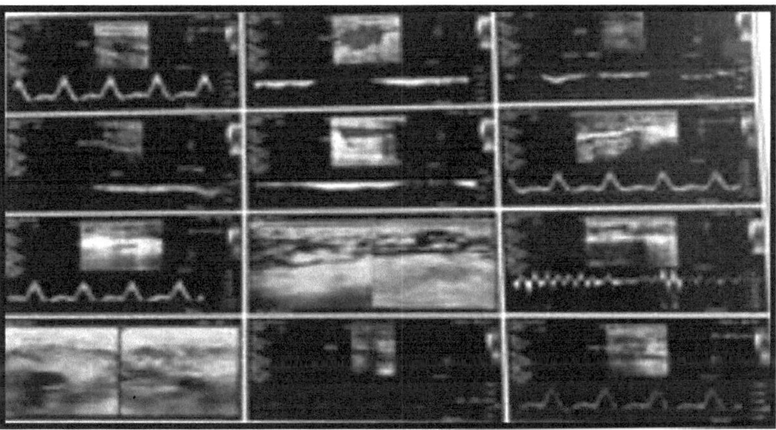

**Venous Doppler of Leg**
**Incompetent Superficial Saphenous Vein**

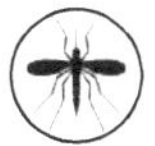

# Diagnosis of CVI

The diagnosis of CVI can be made on clinical grounds alone in the majority of patients. Noninvasive vascular assessment help evaluate alternative pathologic conditions that may mimic venous disease and identify the presence of venous obstruction or reflux. The degree of reflux correlates with the chronicity and size of the venous ulcer.

The ankle/brachial index by vascular Doppler ultrasonography is a useful test for patients with lower extremity ulceration to exclude concomitant arterial disease, which contraindicates the use of compression therapy. This index is unreliable in diabetes, and calcific noncompressible arteries. In these situations, high clinical suspicion of arterial disease must be evaluated. Continuous-wave Doppler studies provide useful anatomic information on the level of obstruction or valvular dysfunction. But it does not distinguish superficial from deep venous insufficiency. Colour flow duplex ultrasound scanning provides the most accurate, reproducible, noninvasive assessment of venous disease. The presence of reflux, obstruction, or a combination of both can be determined.

**Impedance Photoplethysmography**

Impedance Photoplethysmography is a technique that uses optical methods to detect and measure the degree of venous reflux and the efficiency of the calf muscle pump at rest and after exercise occurring in the microvascular bed of tissue. It is a reliable, widely used, noninvasive test to detect deep vein thrombosis (DVT) in the leg(impedance) caused by blood volume variations. The blood volume in the calf distal to the cuff normally increases. However, in DVT, blood volume increases less than expected. This test is especially sensitive for DVT in the popliteal and iliofemoral venous systems. Electrodes from a plethysmograph are applied to the patient's leg to record changes in electrical resistance. Occlusion of the superficial system with a tourniquet will allow assessment of deep venous obstruction with these simple tests.

To perform the test, a light-emitting diode (LED) is placed over the medial ankle region. Transmitted light is reflected in the PPG diode with the intensity of the reflection indicative of the red cell content of the subcutaneous tissues. After establishing a baseline, the patient is asked to perform 10 tiptoe maneuvers or to sequentially perform dorsi and plantar flexion of the ankle 10 times. These maneuvers serve to empty the subcutaneous veins, and the PPG recording decreases from the baseline value. As the veins refill passively, the PPG recording rises back to the baseline value.

In the presence of venous reflux, the veins refill more quickly. A venous refill time (VRT) <20 seconds indicates venous reflux. If an abnormal reflux time is normalized with the application of a superficial tourniquet, isolated superficial reflux is present. If the venous refill time does not normalize, either deep venous reflux or a combination of superficial and deep venous reflux is present.

**Air plethysmography**

Air plethysmography (APG) is a noninvasive physiologic examination that measures relative volume changes in the limb in response to postural changes and muscular activity. The test is more typically used by clinicians who perform large numbers of interventional venous procedures.

APG measures pressure changes in the cuff, which are translatable to volume changes within the leg. The venous volume is measured and used to calculate a venous filling index (VFI). Changes in the volume are measured by air displacement within a polyurethane cuff that is wrapped around the calf and inflated to a preset pressure. The test begins with the patient supine. The limb being evaluated is elevated to drain the venous system. Once the venous system is emptied, the leg volume is recorded and the patient is asked to stand, after which the volume is recorded again. The difference in the recorded leg volume is the functional venous volume. The time needed to fill 90 percent of the functional venous volume is the venous filling time. The venous filling index is functional venous volume divided by the venous filling time; a normal venous filling index is <2 mL/sec. The greater the venous filling index, the more severe the reflux. The residual volume fraction, which is the ratio of the residual volume to the function venous volume, is directly proportional to ambulatory venous pressure, which is used to diagnose venous hypertension. APG primarily provides an overall assessment of venous function but cannot localize sites of venous reflux.

# Medical Treatment of CVI

The treatment of CVI is directed toward the correction of venous hypertension and its adverse effects. The approaches used to provide relief of pain, reduction of edema, control of infection, improvement of lipodermatosclerosis, healing of any ulceration, and prevention of recurrence.

The simple method to counteract the effects of venous hypertension is complete bed rest and leg elevation. Elevation of the affected leg to above the level of the heart for 30 minutes, three or four times per day may be a reasonable protocol for improvement of edema in early venous insufficiency. This is inadequate for advanced venous disease or ulceration. In these patients, compression therapy is indicated. The application of pressure to treat venous insufficiency was known to Hippocrates and practiced in ancient Greece and Rome. Compression raises the local hydrostatic pressure and decreases the superficial venous pressure, thereby reducing the edema. The compression of a normal limb decreases cutaneous blood flow. In contrast, in an edematous extremity, cutaneous blood flow and blood flow in the superficial and deep veins are increased by compression because of the reduction of edema. Lymphatic flow and fibrinolysis also improve with compression and exercise. Compression improves reflux in the deep venous system, render incompetent valves functional, but unfortunately, the hemodynamic benefits of stockings are lost once they are removed. Compression therapy plays a significant role in the management of CVI and ulceration. Its success is directly related to the patient's compliance. Patients careful with their compression therapy have a significantly improved ulcer healing rate and decreased rate of recurrence. More than 90% healing of venous ulceration is possible with a strict regimen of cleansing and elastic compression.

**The compression therapy** for CVI is initially aimed at edema reduction and treatment of ulceration. The maintenance phase is best maintained with graded compression stockings. That is putting maximal pressure at the ankle and minimal at the thigh. An external pressure of 30 to 40 mm Hg at the ankle is necessary to prevent capillary exudation. The initial stage of edema treatment is more effective by using long-stretch (elastic) bandages which provide adequate working pressures and higher resting pressures than rigid bandages do. There are three classes of elastic bandages characterized by increasing degrees of compression. Lightweight (Class-I) and light support (class- II) bandages are used in mild edema and ankle sprains. These are relatively inelastic and rigid. Class-III bandages are compression bandages that may provide up to 40 mm Hg of ankle pressure and are used in the treatment of severe varicosities and severe edema. Multilayered bandages (three or four layers) are easily adapted to legs of various sizes and provide sustained pressures of 40 to 45 mm Hg at the ankle, graded down to 17 mm Hg below the knee. These bandages are effective in healing recalcitrant ulcerations and may, therefore, be more cost-effective because of faster healing rates.

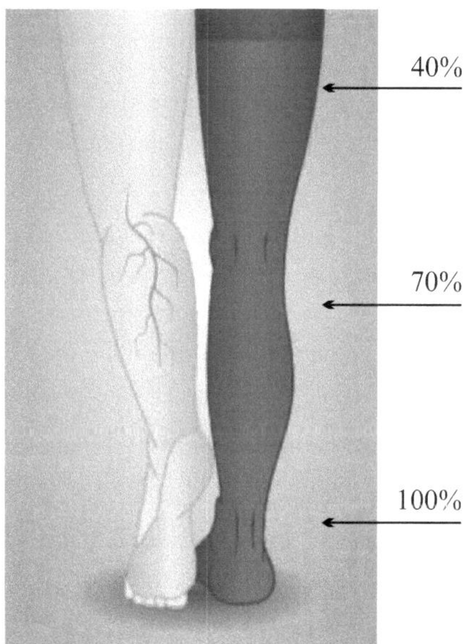


**COMPRESSION STOCKINGS**

Pneumatic compression devices have been used for venous insufficiency. These devices provide intermittent compression and were initially developed for the treatment of lymphedema and deep venous prophylaxis. Unfortunately, they require multiple treatments and sedentary periods. So this approach is effective in bedridden or inactive patients. Compression stocking becomes the mainstay of therapy once venous ulcers are healed. A graded compression stocking is available in four classes.

| Grade | The pressure at the ankle | Indication |
|---|---|---|
| I | 20 to 30 mm Hg | Mild edema |
| II | 30 to 40 mmHg | Severe Varicosities & Moderate edema |
| III | 40 to 50 mmHg | Severe edema & CVI |
| IV | > 60 mmHg | Severe edema & CVI |

Compression stockings should be replaced every six months for optimal effectiveness. Compliance with below-knee garments may be better because they are easier to apply.

**Contraindications of Compression Stocking -** Experts have described several possible contraindications and/or precautions to complete decongestive therapy, and in particular, to manual lymphatic drainage. Although commonly followed, these contraindications are predominantly based upon theoretical concerns, and there are few clinical data to support them.

The complete decongestive therapy for the patients should be made with the guidance of a trained lymphologist and clinician.

Active cellulitis, neoplasm, or other inflammations of the infected limb (complete decongestive therapy may spread the infection or exacerbate symptoms).

Moderate-to-severe heart failure (which may be exacerbated by the increase in central venous volume induced by mobilization of the lymphatic fluid).

Acute deep vein thrombosis (since embolism may result from dislodging of the clot).

Relative contraindications, such that patients may be treated but may warrant monitoring, include:

Uncontrolled hypertension (which may be exacerbated by the increase in central venous blood volume caused by manual lymphatic drainage and compression bandaging). In this case, the patient's cardiac functions are monitored during the treatment phase.

Diabetes mellitus (since associated vasculopathy or neuropathy may decrease the sensing of pain with improperly fitting compression garments, possibly leading to tissue injury and infection).

Limb paralysis (since a flaccid limb may offer insufficient resistance when compression bandages and garments are used, and any decrease in sensation may promote injury from improperly fitting compression garments).

**Pharmacologic therapy**

Diuretics help in fluid mobilization and effective only if used in conjunction with compression therapy. Antimicrobials have been used extensively in the treatment of venous ulceration, even though these wounds are not infected. Bacterial culture of the exudate is the accurate means to determine whether the ulcer is infected or simply colonized and decide the most appropriate antibiotic therapy. Topical antiseptic compounds such as povidone-iodine have been used to treat venous ulcers. The commercially available concentrations are tissue toxic and their routine use retard wound healing. Cadexomer iodine preparations having antimicrobial efficacy, without cellular toxicity decrease ulcer size and healing. Systemic antibiotics are not efficacious in the treatment of venous ulcers and should be reserved for use in complicated cellulitis.

A flavonoid (Daflon) decreases white cell adhesion, reduces capillary permeability and increases red cell velocity. It has some promise in the treatment of small venous ulcerations. Aspirin 300 mg daily has been associated with an increased rate of ulcer healing.

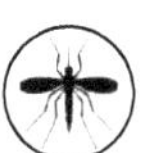

# Surgical Treatment

**Occlusive dressings** wet-to- dry type has been the mainstay of ulcer care due to ease of application and low cost. This technique is painful, causes desiccation of the wound and results in the removal of viable tissue along with necrotic tissue. Occlusive dressings are less painful to remove and provide a moist environment, which permits more rapid wound healing. The types of occlusive dressings available are hydrogels, alginates, hydrocolloids, foams, and films. No available occlusive dressings are superior to a simple, nonadherent dressing placed properly under a compression bandage.

**Sclerotherapy** agents cause endothelial damage by their actions as either osmotic or detergent agents. Osmotic agents achieve their effect by dehydrating endothelial cells through osmosis. Detergents are surface-active agents that damage the endothelium by interfering with cell membrane lipids. Hypertonic saline is an osmotic agent that is commonly used for lower extremity sclerotherapy. Dilutions between 11.7 and 23.4% are used depending on the diameter of the treated vein, with lower concentrations used for narrower veins. Hypertonic saline is frequently mixed with a local anesthetic to reduce the pain associated with injection (20% saline plus 2% lidocaine).

**Saphenous ablation -** Venous reflux in axial veins can be treated with a variety of techniques. For the great saphenous vein, thermal ablation and glue are all associated with higher rates of vein closure (immediate and long term) compared with liquid or foam sclerotherapy.  The rationale used for selecting sclerotherapy to treat the great saphenous vein is based on similar long-term clinical outcomes in the available trials, rather than strictly on rates of vein occlusion. Besides, sclerotherapy is easily repeated since there is no need for general anesthesia. Treatment of other axial veins (small saphenous, accessory saphenous) follows similar principles.

**Perforator ablation -** The presence of reflux in perforator veins following saphenous ablation is known to be a risk factor for nonhealing venous ulcers. Sclerotherapy of perforator veins is associated with fewer complications compared with surgical management of subfascial endoscopic perforator surgery. Ultrasound-guided sclerotherapy of perforator veins reduces the severity of symptoms and signs as determined by venous clinical severity scores.

**Venous Ablation Therapy**

The goals of venous ablation in patients with symptomatic superficial venous disease are improvement in symptoms as well as appearance. Venous ablation is thought to produce beneficial effects by reducing venous volume in the limb and thereby the effects of venous hypertension on the cutaneous tissues.

When combined saphenous and perforator reflux is identified, saphenous reflux is treated first. Perforator reflux often resolves following saphenous ablation. Persistent perforators identified by duplex ultrasound following saphenous ablation can be managed concurrently with phlebectomies as needed, or at a later time with ultrasound-guided sclerotherapy or endovenous methods.

Options - Several venous ablation techniques, including minimally invasive and surgical methods, are available and are classified by their method of vein destruction: chemical, thermal, or nonthermal. Combination treatments have also been described. The choice of most appropriate intervention for superficial vein reflux depends on the size and location of the involved veins. Treatment goals include improvement of symptoms and appearance, reduction of edema, improvement in skin changes, and healing of ulcers.

**Thermal ablation -** Thermal ablation involves the generation of heat at a temperature high enough to denature the proteins that constitute the vein wall. This can be accomplished with radiofrequency energy, or with laser light introduced into the lumen of an incompetent vein (great saphenous, small saphenous). The use of steam has also been described. Because of the need for heat generation to effectively ablate the vein, additional infiltration of the local anesthetic saline mixture is required to reduce pain along the saphenous vein.

**Nonthermal ablation -** Nonthermal ablation techniques are also available. Because there is no heat, nonthermal ablation has the advantage of avoiding any discomfort associated with local anesthesia, and there is a decreased likelihood for adjacent nerve injury.

**Saphenous vein ligation/stripping -** Saphenous vein ligation and division refer to detachment of the great saphenous vein (GSV) through a small oblique groin incision at its confluence with the saphenofemoral junction and common femoral vein. The incision is usually located along the groin crease, and all tributaries at the saphenofemoral junction are ligated. Flush ligation of the GSV at the saphenofemoral junction without narrowing of the femoral vein is performed.

Anatomic limitations for endovenous ablation -

- Chronic or recurrent phlebitis in the target vein.
- Severe tortuosity in which passage of the device may not be possible.
- Target veins that are not at least 1 cm deep to the skin dermis may lead to skin burns.
- Large veins (>1.0 cm) have a high risk of nonclosure.

Contraindications to ablation therapies -

- **Acute deep venous thrombosis** - Endovenous ablation is contraindicated in patients with acute deep vein thrombosis due to the risk of developing a new thrombosis.
- **Superficial vein thrombophlebitis** - Endovenous ablation generally should not be performed in patients who have signs of acute superficial vein thrombosis due to the increased risk of deep venous thrombosis.
- **Pregnancy** - Pregnant patients should defer vein treatments until at least six weeks after delivery due to prothrombotic risk and postpartum hormonal changes.

A compression stocking is advised to wear following sclerotherapy for varicose veins or treatment of reflux continuously for 48 hours after treatment, after which time they may be worn during the day (off at night and to bathe) for next two weeks. Longer duration of compression therapy is required following sclerotherapy for telangiectasis or reticular veins.

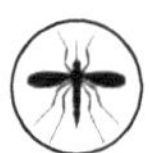

# Conclusion

Lymphedema shares many clinical features with chronic venous insufficiency (CVI). Lymphedema is distinguished from CVI by an absence of typical varicose veins, an absence of characteristic skin change distribution (brawny discoloration at the medial ankle, and alleviation of symptoms and reduction of swelling with limb elevation. Duplex ultrasound can demonstrate typical findings of venous valvular insufficiency. However, a subset of patients with longstanding and severe chronic venous insufficiency may develop concurrent lymphedema. Acute deep venous thrombosis – include acute swelling, pain, and erythema involving one limb. The onset of edema and the associated symptoms of acute erythema, calf pain readily distinguish DVT from lymphedema. Lymphedema is a major cause of disfigurement and disability in endemic areas, leading to significant economic and psychosocial impact. It is the second leading cause of disability worldwide. Chronic lower limb swelling is frequently encountered in clinical practice. Recurrent lymphangitis due to *Wuchereria bancrofti* infection and chronic venous insufficiency is most common. Chronic inflammation and fibrosis are the histological hallmarks of lymphedema leg. Systemic antibiotic therapy and elastic compression stocking are required in both cases. Obstruction of arterial blood flow must be evaluated before advising elastic compression stocking.

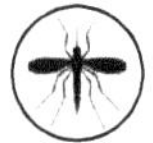

# REFERENCES


1. Greene AK. Epidemiology and morbidity of lymphedema. In: Lymphedema Presentation, Diagnosis, and Treatment, Greene AK, Slavin SA, Brorson H (Eds), Springer, Cham 2015. p.33.

2. Kerchner K, Fleischer A, Yosipovitch G. Lower extremity lymphedema update: pathophysiology, diagnosis, and treatment guidelines. J Am Acad Dermatol 2008; 59:324.

3. U.S. Department of Health & Human Services. Parasites - Lymphatic Filariasis: Epidemiology & Risk Factors. https://www.cdc.gov/parasites/lymphaticfilariasis/epi.html (Accessed on April 02, 2019).

4. International Society of Lymphology. The diagnosis and treatment of peripheral lymphedema: 2013 Consensus Document of the International Society of Lymphology. Lymphology 2013; 46:1.

5. Yasuhara H, Shigemitsu H, Muto T. A study of the advantages of elastic stockings for leg lymphedema. IntAngiol 1996; 15:272.

6. Gloviczki P, Comerota AJ, Dalsing MC, et al. The care of patients with varicose veins and associated chronic venous diseases: clinical practice guidelines of the Society for Vascular Surgery and the American Venous Forum. J VascSurg 2011; 53:2S.

7. Wittens C, Davies AH, Bækgaard N, et al. Editor's Choice - Management of Chronic Venous Disease: Clinical Practice Guidelines of the European Society for Vascular Surgery (ESVS). Eur J VascEndovascSurg 2015; 49:678.

8. Fukaya E, Flores IS, Lindholm D, et al. Clinical and Genetic Determinants of Varicose Veins. Circulation 2018; 138:2869.

9. Van Gent WB, Catarinella FS, Lam YL, et al. Conservative versus surgical treatment of venous leg ulcers: 10-year follow up of a randomized, multicenter trial. Phlebology 2015; 30:35.

10. Kostas TI, Ioannou CV, Drygiannakis I, et al. Chronic venous disease progression and modification of predisposing factors. J VascSurg 2010; 51:900.

11. Eberhard ML, Lammie PJ 1991. Laboratory diagnosis of filariasis. Clin Lab Med 11: 977-1010.

12. Rocha A, Addis D, Ribeiro ME, Norões J, Baliza M, Medeiros Z, Dreyer G 1996. Evaluation of the Og4C3 ELISA in Wuchereria bancrofti infection: infected persons with undetectable or ultra-low microfilarial densities. Trop Med Int Health 1: 859-864.

13. Demirtas Y, Ozturk N, Yapici O, Topalan M. Supermicrosurgically mphaticovenular anastomosis and lymphaticovenous implantation for treatment of unilateral lower extremity lymphedema. Microsurgery 2009; 29:609.

14. Monnin-Delhom ED, Gallix BP, Achard C, et al. High resolution unenhanced computed tomography in patients with swollen legs. Lymphology 2002; 35:121.

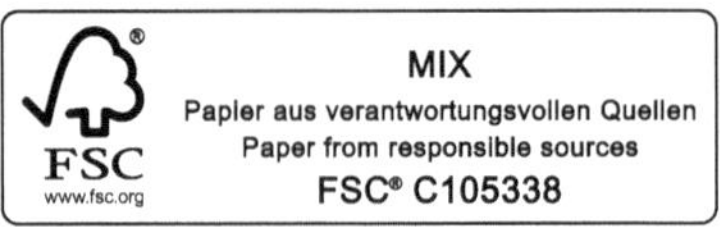

Printed by Books on Demand GmbH, Norderstedt / Germany